Don't Wait, Lose Weight!

Lose Weight without Dieting.
Heal Your Body & Mind.
Healthy Habits, Mindful Eating,
Nutrition Psychology,
Motivation to Weight Loss and so on.

Jolene Daisy

Dedication

I dedicate this book to my family.

Table of Contents

Introduction; Do You Need a Diet to Lose Weight?

Have you ever wondered how many diets there are? It turns out that their number is measured in thousands. These are various mono-diets (on kefir, buckwheat and other products), low-carb diets, protein diets, Mediterranean, Japanese, Hollywood, etc. Why are there so many? Variety is so great because there is no ideal diet that would suit absolutely everything. Most diets have contraindications, it is better to consult the doctor before starting the diet so as not to harm your health. Often, people, wanting to quickly lose weight, go on some fast-fashionable diet, succumbing to advertising. Indeed, there are quick ways to lose weight for several days or weeks, but that weight is gained again as people start to eat in their usual manner. Is that familiar to you? I think yes. Most people at least once in their lives were on a diet with the goal of losing weight.

How do you find a solution to the problem? How do you lose weight forever and without harm to health? I have good news for you: losing weight without diet is possible! But a miracle cannot happen too quickly. Therefore, this will take time and a great desire to be slim, healthy and beautiful. Let's take the first step on the way to a beautiful figure!

1. Mindful Eating is the Key to Health

Are your thoughts busy at the time you eat? Perhaps during a meal, you scroll in your head talking to your boss or a friend, reading a newspaper or watching TV? It's no secret that many people do so. Some time management guidelines recommend that during the morning coffee, you make a work plan for the day or view business correspondence. Maybe from the position of time management, this will save you valuable time, but is your own health not more expensive? From the standpoint of healthy eating, it is absolutely unacceptable to eat in a hurry, to eat on the run or to skip breakfast. If you decide to drink coffee in the morning, then allow yourself to enjoy its taste and aroma. And when you begin to work, give yourself to the work. Otherwise, you can miss the taste of life itself.

In general, mindfulness is the ability to live in the present moment i.e. to live in the here and now. The most important tools of awareness are attention and observation. Why is attention so important? That object or process, on which our attention stops, is firmly imprinted in our consciousness. Consciousness always goes for attention; therefore, our emotions, thoughts, actions, and, ultimately, our energy are directed towards our consciousness.

Everyone knows that the food that gets into our stomach nourishes our physical body. However, few people thought about why it is important to feel the taste of food, to inhale the fragrance, to receive visual information about its appearance. The fact is that these impressions nourish our subtle body energy. When you read while eating or vice-versa, then your mind and energy, as well as your attention, are directed first to the assimilation of what you are reading. Your subtle body receives information and emotions from what you are reading as food. On the digestion of food impressions, energy is not directed; the feeling of enjoying food is therefore lost. At the physical level, the digestive gland is inhibited as well as the secretion of gastric juices. As a result, the whole process of digestion is disrupted. This inevitably could lead to conditions such as gastritis, diabetes, and obesity. I hope now you understand why it is not advisable for you to read, watch TV or read your mail while eating. It's all about attention and energy.

So, the first thing to do is to stop taking food mechanically and learn how to enjoy eating. In the families of our ancestors, there was a tradition: the utterance of a Thanksgiving prayer before a meal. I think that very few people do this today. Prayer before eating was a kind of ritual, allowing the body to tune in for food. We smell, we contemplate the food, but we do not hurry to absorb it, we first tune into the process. At this point, the anxiety associated with food recedes. It is noticed that the rituals before eating make the meal tastier, and the food is better absorbed. Try to invent your own ritual; maybe you would prefer to light a candle or serve the table beautifully, even if you eat alone. Or you will eat using Chinese chopsticks. Think about the fact that food becomes a part of us, and we are a part of the Universe. Turning the process of food into a ritual, we feel a connection with the universal spirit that permeates all that exists. People may object to this, as in this age of high speeds it is not always possible to precede food by ritual, there is simply not enough time for it. I will answer this: even if you are a very busy person and usually your business lunch takes place at the nearest cafe to the office, you can still at least mentally before the meal, thank the universe for the food sent to you. Just feel the power of gratitude to the present moment!

"The whole banquet is in the first spoonful" – this is how the wizard Merlin taught. Of course, he talked about spiritual knowledge, but as an example, he took a bowl of soup. Indeed, the first spoon in eating is the most important. Do not swallow it quickly, even if you are very hungry. You must feel the food, enjoy and be satisfied with it before you start eating. So, food is an intimate process. Haste here is therefore inappropriate. We must develop the habit of eating slowly, chewing food carefully. When already in the mouth food should become "liquid".

If you usually eat in the company of family, friends or colleagues, you probably know, at least on an intuitive level, that a joint eating unites people. The dining table is a place where relations are "fueled", and a mutual exchange of spirit warmth takes place. An atmosphere of mutual trust and consent is created. Remember the evangelical "breaking bread", when we eat, our minds are open, so during meals it is not recommended to discuss contentious issues, or talk about bad things. Do not eat with people who are easily irritated. Any showdown must be postponed for later, after the meal. If someone at the table thinks about something other than good food, for example, problems in the office or in relationships with friends, it means that he misses the present moment and the enjoyment of eating. You can correct the situation by returning your attention to food. Easy, friendly conversation, usually arising at the end of the meal or at the stage of its completion, is the best seasoning for your food.

2. Feeling of Hunger: Should We Fight It?

How much do you usually eat? How often do you eat? What does your diet consist of? You should answer honestly to these questions because a conscious eating is an understanding of what exactly, how much and when you eat. Let's try to understand these questions together.

Ideally, you should eat when hunger is felt. But here lies the danger, the first urge to run to the fridge and quickly grab something that can be eaten without cooking or with minimal processing, is not wise. This is the habit of many people who are overweight. How do you take control of the feeling of hunger and whether it should be done? Of course, if you are the master of your body, you must control it, and therefore you must learn to control your appetite and weight. If you are a slave to your stomach, then ... No, I do not want to consider this option. People are not born as slaves. Definitely – you are the master of your life and your body.

If you think that your appetite is pathologically overestimated, be sure to undergo a medical examination. Perhaps, you have violations in the work of the endocrine or digestive system. So, if you have a dysbacteriosis, then aligning the bacterial background, you will get rid of the problem and normalize your appetite. It happens that the feeling of hunger is associated with psychological problems, in which case you may need the help of a psychologist. So, hormonal glitches, the use of antibiotics, hormonal pills can influence the increase in appetite. But let's talk about other cases.

Suddenly, the most powerful stimulant for increasing appetite is a diet. The body perceives your rejection of certain products as a threat to your existence. The brain then automatically turns on an auto-save program and increases the feeling of hunger. The deficiency of vitamins, minerals, amino acids, and macronutrients also strengthen hunger.

Frequent meals in small portions, as a rule, do not bring the desired results. With such eating, the walls of the stomach do not stretch, so the brain does not associate a snack with a full meal. Because the brain does not receive a saturation signal, you experience an almost constant feeling of hunger. Therefore, it makes no sense to eat more often than 6 times a day. The optimal number of meals is 4-5 times a day, including snacks.

Between meals, you need to occupy yourself with something that brings you pleasure: it could be an interesting occupation, work or hobby, as well as communication with friends. This very well reduces appetite, moderates exercise, walking, and meditation. A glass of water will also help to muffle the raging appetite. When life is interesting and saturating, then food recedes into the background.

Friendly advice: every time before opening the fridge for a snack, do 5 sit-ups. Appetite decreases – it is checked. -)

3. How Much to Eat?

Let's talk about the size of the portion. I think that you have already heard about the rule of hands in the diet (not to be confused with the rules of the hands for electromagnetism -). You have to eat at once as much, as it fits in the palms of your hands. This volume corresponds to the size of your stomach and is sufficient for saturation. Put the food on your plate, evaluate visually, whether it fits in your palms. You can eat a little less, but not more. Remember that the feeling of satiety does not come immediately; the satiety signal comes to the brain about 30 minutes after eating. People, who have learned not to overeat, and have made it the norm, live longer.

Many people, who want to lose weight, start a nutrition diary. Some use an ordinary paper notebook for this, some use Microsoft Excel and

Google Drive cloud. In the diary it is necessary to indicate the meal time (beginning and ending), the amount of food eaten in grams and its caloric value. To determine the latter you need to print the calorie tables of the main food products and put them on the first page of your diary. It is also useful to write in the diary such information: where and with whom did you eat, why you took food (hunger, boredom, eat up after the child, etc.), evaluate your taste sensations. If during the day everything is impossible to record, then you can photograph food and make quick notes on your mobile phone, and in the evening, you can rewrite. Maintaining such a diary will help you to understand your eating habits and take measures to correct them.

To calculate the daily requirement for calories, there are special calorie calculator programs. Remember: a person eats to live. If your body does not spend all the calories received, you begin to gain weight. We need to find a middle way in which your body has enough energy for life and nothing superfluous is stored up. If you want to lose weight, you can slightly reduce the amount of calories consumed or increase their consumption. But we must do this without violence against our body.

4. Nutritional Habits: What to Eat to Lose Weight?

Here we smoothly turn to talk about which products should be preferred. How to lose weight without starving? If you set a target to lose weight, then when choosing products for your menu, pay attention not only to calorie content but also to the content of protein, fat and carbohydrate foods. At the right approach to nutrition, caloric intake should be reduced by reducing the amount of fast carbohydrates (they have a sweet taste and a high glycemic index: such as sweet carbonated drinks, cookies, candies and other sweets and pastries). Also, you should stop eating excessive amounts of fat. At the same time, proteins must enter the body in the required amount. This is because proteins contain lipotropic substances that promote fat burning and, at moderate physical exertion, activate metabolic processes and maintain muscle mass. Let's take a closer look at what foods you need to eat to lose weight without starving:

- ✓ Products containing protein, which is the main building material of our body. This is a low-fat chicken breast, lean beef or turkey meat, fish and seafood.
- ✓ Complex carbohydrates: fresh vegetables (especially cabbage, sweet pepper, carrots),

macaroni from coarse flour, buckwheat, brown rice.
- ✓ Of the fats, it is preferable to use olive oil of a high degree of purification.
- ✓ Fresh fruits rich in vitamins: green apples, grapefruits, oranges.
- ✓ Low-fat dairy products: yogurts, low-fat cottage cheese.
- ✓ Limit the use of salt.
- ✓ As a snack, you can use nuts: almonds or walnuts. But we must remember that nuts have a high fat content, so they can be consumed no more than 20 grams per day.
- ✓ Green tea (helps to eliminate toxins).

As you can see, the choice of food is great enough. You definitely do not have to complain about diversity and starve. From these products, you can make for yourself an excellent menu!

When you begin to eat right, then be surprised by the changes that will happen to you. You will feel better, you will have the energy for work and creativity, and also, the diseases will recede. Over time, your body develops the habit of eating properly and eating healthy food. You will not want to look at popcorn, fried potatoes, chicken nuggets, sausages and other unhealthy products. Believe me; eating habits are very important for a person. Man is what he eats. Just remember that habits are developed over the years; they often come from your childhood, so in many cases, it can be difficult to change your habits in an instant. The main thing is your decision to start eating right, do not despair in case of breakdowns and temporary setbacks, move forward and do not stop. I believe you will succeed!

5. Listen to Your Body!

Your body is your friend, and you must learn how to listen to it.

First, you need to learn to recognize during the meal, the moment when you are full. When you are comfortable with what you have eaten, there is no feeling of overeating. The body gives you a signal - enough has been eaten, it's time to stop!

Secondly, listen to the feeling of hunger and learn to distinguish true hunger from false. Eat only when really hungry.

Thirdly, listen to what your body wants at the moment: hot or cold, meat or vegetables, cereal or fruit. Build your diet to suit the needs of the body.

6. The Reason of Overweight is in Your Head: the Psychological Causes of Excess Weight

So, you made a decision to lose weight, began to eat properly, and excluded harmful foods from the diet? Your hormone levels and blood sugar are normal, but for some reason, the weight does not want to decrease? What's the matter? Really, the causes of excess weight should be sought not only in improper nutrition or in insufficient physical activity. All problems are generated by the mind. In most cases, overweight is only a symptom, a manifestation of various internal problems. The way to an ideal figure is often blocked by psychological barriers: fears, avoiding problems, perfectionism, emotional states. Let's talk about typical psychological problems and ways to solve them.

Many problems come from childhood. Did your parents praise you for your good appetite? Force you to eat all that was in the plate, until the last crumb? Blackmailed you with sweets, trying to get you to eat dinner? Encouraged by sweets for good behavior? They used tasty food as comfort or entertainment, like "if you eat candy or a cake, you will become more cheerful and sadness will pass"? The child tries to be good, to deserve the praise of parents, obediently eats, although already full. So gradually the habit of overeating is formed and the orientation toward hunger as the main reason for food intake is lost. Becoming adults, many people unconsciously copy their parents, their lifestyle and eating habits.

Overweight often appears from the inability to cope with your emotions. According to Eastern philosophy, emotions feed our subtle body. If during the day we experienced a lot of different emotions, then our subtle body is full, and the physical body, on the contrary, reduces appetite. It happens when we are overtaken by love, or a creative breakthrough, or vivid impressions on the journey, or a meeting with an interesting person. We are so pleased to experience positive emotions! About food in this case, even when there is no time to think, negative emotions are often suppressed in us, and this is fraught with consequences. It happens that the working day turned out to be nervous, you could not cope with the negativity in any situation, and then all evening you slam the refrigerator door all the time. Eastern philosophy defines this as an example of energy indigestion. This is when a person tries to compensate for undigested energy food with physical food. Psychology says that people tend to engage in emotional eating. Stress, loss of loved ones, loneliness, dissatisfaction, irritation, and boredom can lead to overweight, especially if a person does not have enough support, or an opportunity to express emotions.

How to be? We must learn to control ourselves, manage our emotions, and give them a constructive way out. Now I will return to the issue of awareness. Either you learn to be aware of your emotions and control them, or emotions will start to control you. Emotional awareness will help you communicate candidly and effectively. It would help you make wise decisions, and also build strong and healthy relationships. If you were offended and you are smothered in tears – you can cry, it will become easier. If the anger is boiling, you can beat a pear in the gym or shout loudly in the forest. If you are bored – do the cleaning in your house. It's better than slamming the refrigerator door in search of food. But remember that this is not a solution to the problem or situation that caused such emotions to begin with.

Oftentimes, overweight people unconsciously pursue secondary benefits. For example, a person is afraid of building relationships, so he does not want to seem attractive to the opposite sex. The wife gets rid of her husband's jealousy, growing fat and becoming less attractive. The boss raises his authority due to his massive figure. In these cases, fat is a kind of protection. It seems that in words there is a desire to lose weight, but in fact, a person does not want and is actually even afraid to lose weight. Just be honest with yourself.

In fact, the reasons why people do not want to part with excess weight even more, for example, is a sense of guilt and low self-esteem. Here you must learn to forgive yourself and love yourself. In many cases, a person can realize problems and work on themselves, but sometimes a qualified psychologist can be of help.

7. Motivate Yourself to Lose Weight!

Can you answer the question, why do you want to lose weight? Maybe you want to get into a fashionable dress or your favorite jeans? Well, I think it will be enough to quickly lose 7-8 pounds in a week. This can be done quickly, but not for long as the case may be. Or maybe you want to look like a top model or be slimmer than your girlfriend? It's unlikely that it will work because comparing yourself to other people is not right. Comparison generates a rivalry that can grow into envy or jealousy. Even if you have a healthy rivalry, without signs of envy, you need to remember that all people are different. Comparing yourself with others limits your potential, and also deprives you of uniqueness. Do not constantly compare yourself with other people, be yourself! You can compare yourself today with yourself yesterday. If you have your photo, where you are in the form desired for you, put it on your table, let it be your incentive. It will be easier to lose weight if you are conscious of that overweight which is harmful to your health. It obstructs the active way of life that you are striving for. Think about your personal motivation (feel the ease of movement, get rid of complexes, etc.) and motivate yourself correctly. The right motives for losing weight are always connected with changing oneself and one's lifestyle.

Consciousness, volition, and intention are links of one chain, allowing us to activate our energy and directing it to the transformation of our body and consciousness. People with a high level of consciousness have a strong volition, they're able to set goals and achieve them. You, too, can form a firm intention to lose those excess pounds, if you certainly realize that it is vitally important for you.

A few tips for those who want to lose weight:

- ✓ Determine exactly what weight you want to possess. This digit should constantly flicker in your mind, and it is better to write it down on a piece of paper. But do not set the bar high, set yourself a real task.

- ✓ Imagine how you will look and feel after you reach your goal and lose excess weight, and become active and healthy. Consider yourself in detail, what your body looks like, and feel what emotions you are experiencing. Concentrate on these images in the evening, when you go to bed and in the morning, being between a dream and a reality.

✓ Love and respect yourself no matter what the scales show. Remember that you can effectively lose weight only with a positive attitude.

8. Drink Water and Lose Weight!

I think you know that the human body mostly consists of water. All metabolic processes in the body occur in the aquatic environment. Drinking water improves metabolism, promotes the proper absorption of nutrients and the removal of toxins. Ageing is the drying of the body i.e. it is the reducing of the amount of water in its cells and tissues. During a day, a person should drink about two liters of clean water. Remember that water most effectively helps to lose weight only when it replaces all other drinks.

It is believed that it is right to drink water immediately after a morning awakening, 1-2 glasses. It is useful to develop the habit of drinking a glass of water 15-20 minutes before eating. This helps reduce appetite and triggers metabolic processes in the body. Drink water when you feel like drinking. Drink water when you feel like eating and be healthy.

Do not forget to note in your food diary how many glasses of water you drank in a day.

9. About the Benefits of a Healthy Sleep.

Scientists came to the conclusion that the less you sleep the more fat you can gain. Sleep plays an important role in maintaining hormones responsible for hunger and making you feel full. A short duration of sleep leads to a higher level of the hormone that causes appetite (leptin) while reducing the concentration of the hormone saturation (ghrelin). Those who want to lose weight should adhere to the sleep regime, the duration of which should be 7-8 hours a day. Try to fall asleep from 22:00 to 24:00. At this time, the body is recovering energy.

10. Physical Activity

Do you think you can lose weight while lying on the couch? Probably, it is possible. With a negative balance of calories, a person will lose weight, but the organism, first of all, will not start to get rid of fat, but of muscle tissue. The body starts to save energy, namely muscles make the maximum contribution to our energy costs. How to lose weight properly? My advice: do not create a caloric deficit of more than 10-20%. Let the speed of such weight loss not be too high (5-6 pounds per month), but your body will not experience a lot of stress. At this time it is useful to give yourself moderate cardio workouts to maintain muscle tone. Walk more, ride a bicycle etc. Physical loads help to increase spending energy and speed up all metabolic processes, but the main thing is to keep your muscle tissue toned. Think about what kind of physical activity you like. It is one thing when you make an effort, working in the gym for a beautiful figure and quite another thing when you are doing what you enjoy and brings the joy of movement. You just have to find the kind of physical activity that you like. Try the swimming pool or tennis court, Nordic walking, yoga or oriental dances – you will not know until you try.

Proper nutrition, regimen, physical activity – all these are the foundation of a happy life. Strong health implies a good state of mind. Thus, everything in the world is interconnected, one supplements another. Focus on changing your lifestyle.

Appendix A; Natural Means for Weight Loss and Clarification of an Organism

In conclusion, I would like to remind readers of the well-known, but perhaps forgotten, ways to lose weight.

Fresh juices

For example, 1 glass of carrot fresh juice on an empty stomach 30 minutes before breakfast will improve digestion and adjust the intestine.

Flax seeds

Flax seeds are rich in amino acids, vitamins and are very useful for the female body. In the stomach, flax seeds swell and envelop the mucous membrane of the stomach, preventing the absorption of fat. This reduces appetite and gives a feeling of satiety. Also, flax seeds have a laxative effect, as in addition, toxins and slags are excreted from the intestine along with feces. Metabolism is thus accelerated. Therefore, the benefits of flax seeds for weight loss are beyond doubt.

Seeds of flax serve as an excellent additive to many dishes. Dry flaxseed for several grams (5-10 gram) can be added to yogurts, kefir, and salads. During the day, you can eat no more than 50 grams (3 tablespoons) of dry flaxseed.

Linseed decoction for weight loss

2 tablespoons of flax seeds can be poured 500 ml boiling water. This is then infused for 2 hours. Take 3 times a day, 100 ml each for 10 days. Then take a break for another 10 days. Flax has a diuretic effect, so it can't be used for cholelithiasis, pancreatitis, or ulcers.

Beetroot salad

1 boiled beetroot to grate on a large grater, fill with 1 tablespoon of vegetable oil. If desired, you can add 1 crushed walnut.

"Broom" salad

For the preparation of salad, fresh carrots, beets, cabbage, and apple are required in equal proportions. These are all grated on a coarse grater. A tablespoon of vegetable oil is added and if desired, a few drops of lemon juice. Do not salt. As a sauce, you can also use kefir with a low percentage of fat.

Salad "Broom" is very useful for constipation and high cholesterol. This will make the colon work, and lightness will appear throughout the body. Salad is contraindicated in the pathologies of the gallbladder, kidneys, gastritis with high acidity, type II diabetes, and flatulence.

Appendix B; Example Food Diary

Food Diary

Day _________ Water _________ 🥛🥛🥛🥛🥛🥛🥛

Breakfast [time_____________]	amount	calories
Snack [time_____________]	amount	calories
Lunch [time_____________]	amount	calories
Snack [time_____________]	amount	calories
Dinner [time_____________]	amount	calories
Snack [time_____________]	amount	calories
Daily Total